First published 2007

Published by
Professor Grace Dorey
Old Hill Farm, Portmore, Barnstaple, Devon, EX32 0HR, UK
Telephone: +44 (0) 1271 321721
Email: grace.dorey@virgin.net
www.yourpelvicfloor.co.uk

ISBN 978-0-9545393-4-4

Love Your Gusset

This little book is for women of all ages.
With a light-hearted approach to a taboo
subject it aims to help women learn to
love their pelvic floor. Just a few simple
daily exercises can make an amazing
difference. Using your pelvic floor muscles
at the right time can help you achieve
orgasm. It can also help to stop those
little leaks when you laugh or sneeze.
It's a delicate subject but, with half of
all women suffering urinary leakage at
some point in their lives, it's worth talking
about. So sit back and have a giggle – but
don't forget to tighten your pelvic floor
muscles first!

Grace Dorey

Contents

Gussets have feelings
Gussets like fun
Stimulate your gusset

Section 4: Gussets and babies

Why it's important to exercise before childbirth
Will exercising my gusset make childbirth difficult?
Why it's important to exercise after childbirth

Section 5: Problem gussets

Help! Things keep falling out!
Dashing to the loo?
My gusset is weak at the back
I need to wear a pad
Restrictions for floppy gussets
Restrictions for prolapsed gussets
Painful gussets
Constipated gussets

Section 4: Loving your gusset

Washing your gusset
Dress up your gusset
Does smoking affect the health of my gusset?
If I am overweight will my gusset sag more?
Love your gusset

What is a gusset?

Take a look in your knickers. What do you see? There are all sorts of interesting things happening down there. Now take them off and look again. What do you see now? There should be a small piece of material in the crotch bit. That's it - the gusset. Small but important, it is supposed to make your panties more comfortable. According to the clever people at the Oxford English Dictionary, a gusset is a 'triangular piece of material let into a garment to strengthen or to enlarge some part in order to give freedom of movement'. So that's that then.

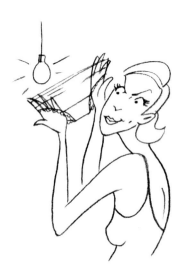

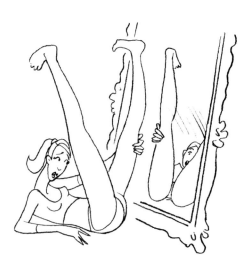

Discover your gusset

Unsurprisingly, your body also has a gusset. Grab a mirror and have a look. The area between your pubes (or front bottom if you're a Brazilian kind of a girl) and your tail bone at the back (where that funny little dimple is) is your gusset. It is also known as your pelvic floor. All the interesting stuff is here, and includes your clitoris (sexual organ), your urethra (your wee hole), your vagina and your anus (your poo hole). Everybody has a gusset and everybody's gusset is different. If you haven't ever thought much about it before, now is the time to start. Let's fall in love with our gussets.

Your gusset has muscles

There are some very important muscles in your gusset. Their job is to stop everything inside you from falling out. How else do you suppose it stays up there? In your gusset you'll also find sphincters. These are the muscles that stop your bladder and bottom from leaking, especially when you are exerting yourself. For women this can be particularly important – especially when laughing. When your pelvic floor muscles are working properly you should be able to control your bladder and bowels, as well as any unexpected parps.

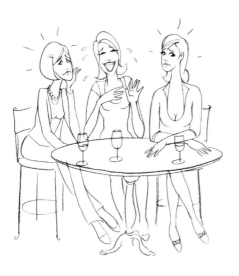

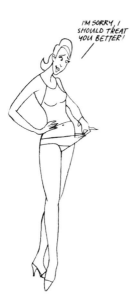

Your gusset has feelings

Don't think that because it has an unsavoury name means it doesn't have feelings too. In fact, your gusset is jam packed with sensory nerves. They are the ones that make you feel all warm and wobbly during sex. There are others that don't have such interesting things to do but are still vital. These nerves allow you to feel when you are peeing and having a poo - hopefully they'll also let you know when you're about to release unwanted wind. But it's not all fun: these same nerves are responsible for the unpleasant dragging sensations you'll feel if you have a prolapse (descent of the vaginal wall) or severe pain if your muscles cramp up.

When gussets go numb

Sometimes you might find that your gusset goes numb. Mostly it means that you have squashed your gusset's nerves. See, we told you that your gusset has feelings. The most common cause of this is from sitting on hard things for too long, like riding a bike with a hard saddle. Ouch. The simple remedy for this is to stand up for a bit or get off your bike and walk for a while. Sometimes gussets can be numb all the time. This is bad and may mean that you may have trapped a nerve in your spine. If you have a constantly numb gusset, do it a favour, take it to see your GP.

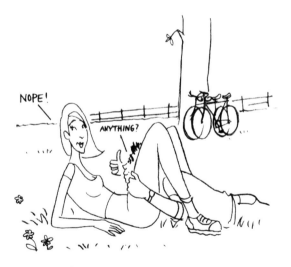

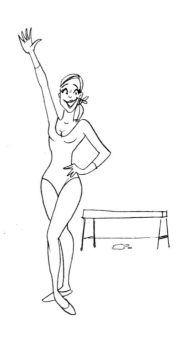

Stretching your gusset

Your gusset is pretty clever. It will let you do the splits and high kicks if you want to - but it's important that it gets the same amount of exercise as the rest of you. Gymnasts sometimes find that, despite having well developed bodies that are able to do all sorts of amazing gymnastic things, their pelvic floor lets them down. This may be due to hypermobility or it may be because they haven't tuned up their gusset to the same level as the rest of them. The result can be untimely leakage. Nobody wants that during a cartwheel on the high bar.

Droopy gusset? You are not alone

If your pelvic floor muscles are weak, they will sag and give you problems when you stand up for a long time. Weak pelvic floor muscles can also cause you to leak when you least expect it. Whilst you might be able to cope with a little dribble after a funny story, when it gets more serious it's no laughing matter. And, worst of all, you may find it more difficult to reach orgasm. It's amazing to think, but almost half of all women suffer from urinary leakage. So you really are not alone. They just aren't telling you they have problems too. Take your gusset to see a Specialist Continence Physiotherapist or Continence Nurse Specialist. They know about this kind of thing and will examine you gently and help you get over it.

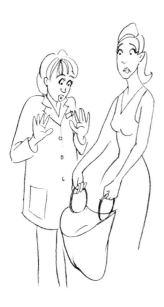

Section 2: Strengthening your gusset

Put your gusset to the test

The first step on the road to gusset loveliness is to check how strong it is. This can be done by trying the Thumb Squeeze Test. As the name suggests you will need a thumb and a gusset to perform this test. It can be done anywhere but we wouldn't recommend doing it on the bus and it's often best to start with your own thumb. It's very easy to perform: place your thumb gently into your vagina. Tighten your muscles by imagining there is a lift inside you. Can you feel them tightening? That's good. The more you exercise your pelvic floor muscles (more about that later) the more you'll feel your muscles getting firmer every time you do the thumb test.

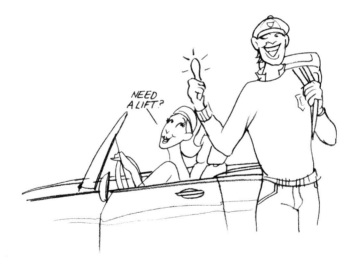

Getting a healthy gusset

A healthy gusset is one that is strong enough to stop your insides from falling out and will keep all your excretive fluids where they should be until you want to get rid of them. It should also be able to relax. Doing pelvic floor exercises will make your gusset stronger and healthy and happy and will improve the blood supply down there, so helping to keep the tissues healthy. And there are other benefits too - a healthy gusset can provide a snug fit for a penis and can enhance all kinds of sexual excitement. And that's worth working for.

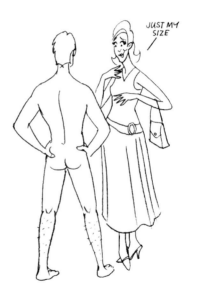

JUST MY
SIZE

Pelvic floor exercises – the secret to a happy gusset

This is the really important bit. Are you sitting comfortably? OK. Now tighten the muscles in your back passage as if you are trying to stop some unwanted gas from escaping. Now tighten the muscles at the front as if you are stopping peeing. Now pull up from the back and front together. Got it? Well done, you have just done a pelvic floor contraction. Now try contracting again and hold it for as long as you can - but not more than 10 seconds. Try not to pull a face and make sure you keep breathing. Then relax. Now you're well on your way to a happy healthy gusset.

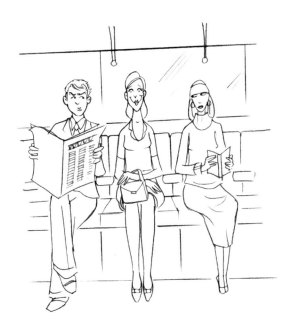

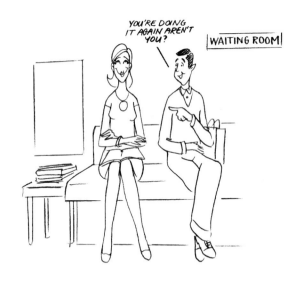

Every day in every way I am getting stronger…

Now you've mastered the pelvic floor contraction you can move on to doing regular exercises. These will make your gusset even stronger. You only need to perform pelvic floor exercises twice a day, but make sure every muscle contraction is as strong as possible. You can perform these exercises in lying, sitting and standing. Perform 3 contractions in each of these positions holding each contraction for no more than 10 seconds. That's only 18 contractions a day. Soon you'll be able to win Gold at the Gusset Olympics!

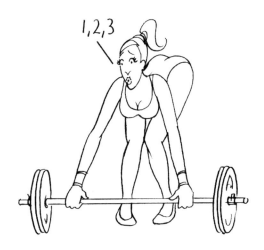

Tighten your gusset during exertion

Importantly, you should be able to tighten your pelvic floor muscles before and during strenuous activities. These 'activities' include coughing, sneezing, laughing, shouting, rising from sitting, pushing and pulling and, of course, lifting. If you can't do this or you can't tighten your muscles at all – and exercises aren't helping – do the right thing by your gusset and treat it to a visit to a Specialist Continence Physiotherapist or Continence Nurse Specialist. They will understand your problem and can help.

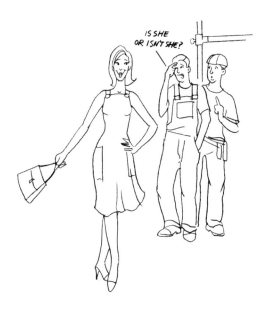

Walk the walk

A good exercise can be to tighten your pelvic floor muscles slightly every time you stand or walk about. After all, these muscles are designed to support your pelvic organs and need to work every time you are upright, however long that is. Once you get used to doing it, it will become a habit. It's great for your posture and no one will know you're doing it.

Section 3: Sexy gussets

A finer vagina

Pelvic floor muscle exercises are also designed to strengthen the muscles that are important for sexual activity. These exercises bring more blood to the pelvic area to help to get you aroused and importantly help you to achieve orgasm. Your orgasm will last longer if your gusset muscles are fit. And that has to be worth working for.

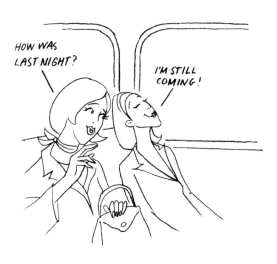

Painful sexual intercourse

If penetration is painful you can try a lubricant. Oestrogen cream may help ladies who experience vaginal dryness. If you have pain when your partner is thrusting you should tell him and ask to change your position better still just do it – he'll think you're going for an Olympic record. However you deal with it, do not put up with pain. If you go on top you can control the depth of penetration. Alternatively you can always ask him to wear a bagel!

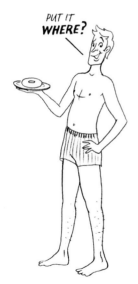

Pain preventing sexual intercourse

Some women avoid sexual intercourse because it is too painful. It's only natural to avoid what hurts you. And it can be a vicious circle, because you tense up if you are expecting penetration to hurt. Having tense muscles will make the pain worse. And so on. A Specialist Continence Physiotherapist can help you to relax these muscles and a Sexual Counsellor can help you with relationship issues.

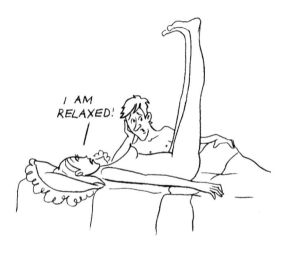

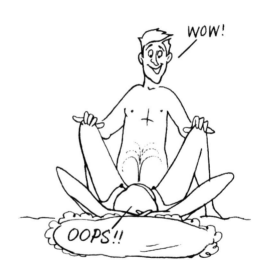

Gussets can leak during intercourse

A lot of women find that they leak a bit during sexual intercourse. The simple answer is to make sure you practise your pelvic floor exercises. It can also help to confide in your partner and empty your bladder before sexual activity. Some men are turned on by this total abandonment. There are whole websites devoted to it. They think it is a female ejaculation!

Gussets have feelings

There are many sensory nerves in your gusset, especially around your clitoris. The clitoris is an organ which has a central glans and divides like a wishbone either side of the vagina for 5-9cm. It becomes swollen with blood during sexual stimulation and your vagina becomes moist. The feelings in your gusset during sexual activity are further enhanced by thoughts of love, fantasy and erotic excitement.

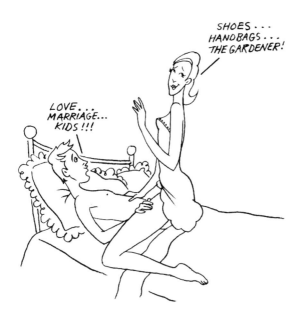

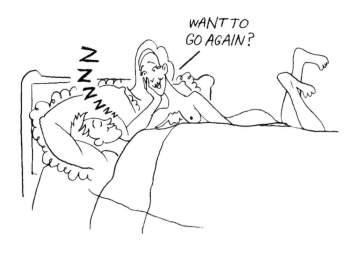

Gussets like fun

When the moment is right, gussets like to be touched, stroked, kissed and stimulated. Anything goes. Every gusset likes different things. The level of stimulation required to reach orgasm is different for everybody. At orgasm your pelvic floor muscles will contract rhythmically. After a short rest you may find that with a bit more stimulation you can achieve another orgasm or even multiple orgasms if your pelvic floor muscles are in good shape.

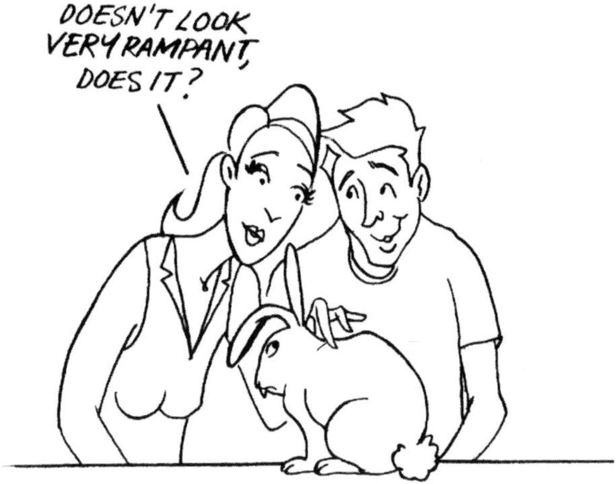
DOESN'T LOOK VERY RAMPANT, DOES IT?

Stimulate your gusset

If you feel comfortable with your own sexuality and your own needs, you will know what stimulation you need when you are with your partner and how to guide him to the spot. You may find that you can gently hold a vibrator over your clitoris to achieve orgasm or you may find that you respond better by using a vaginal vibrator. Of course you can always use a vibrator with your partner – they aren't just for solo sessions you know.

Section 4: Gussets and babies

Why it's important to exercise before childbirth

Pregnancy is going to put some pretty heavy strain on your gusset. Brings tears to your eyes just thinking about it doesn't it? The good news is that having a well exercised pelvic floor will mean the muscles are healthier and firmer and therefore more able to get back into shape after childbirth.

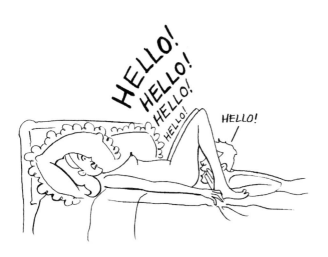

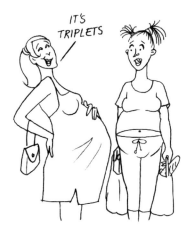

Will exercising my gusset make childbirth difficult?

Exercising your pelvic floor muscles before your delivery does not mean that you will be muscle bound and that the birth will be more difficult. Healthy fit muscles also have the ability to relax to allow the passage of your baby.

Why it's important to exercise after childbirth

After childbirth make sure you get your gusset back into shape by doing some pelvic floor exercises. If your partner complains about being able to drive a bus through your vagina after childbirth you have two choices: get a man with a bigger fella or do some pelvic floor exercises.

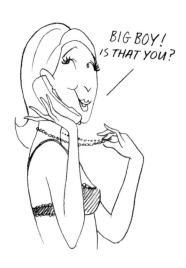

Section 5: Problem gussets

Help! Things keep falling out!

If you use tampons your pelvic floor muscles should be able to keep them in place without any effort on your part. But if you do find that tampons fall out don't panic. It is usually a sign that your gusset may need a bit of work but it's not the end of the world. Strengthening your pelvic floor muscles will help.

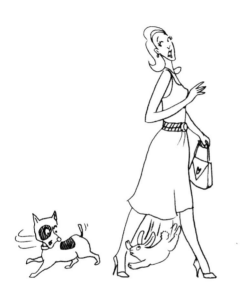

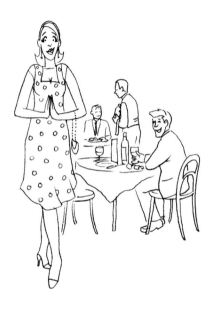

Dashing to the loo?

If you have a desperate urge to visit the toilet, when you rush you may leak urine on the way. Less haste more speed is the key. If you stand still or sit down and relax for one minute until the urge has disappeared your brain can take control. When the strong urge has gone you can walk calmly to the toilet without leaking.

My gusset is weak at the back

Some women experience leakage of faeces and soiling of underwear. They may also find they cannot control their wind. A balanced diet can help to keep your poo nicely formed. Pelvic floor exercises can help to tighten up the anal sphincter and the surrounding pelvic floor muscles. After having a poo, tighten up the muscles in your back passage to return any unpassed faeces back up above the pelvic floor muscles.

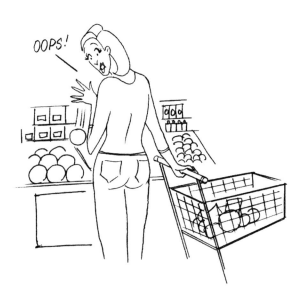

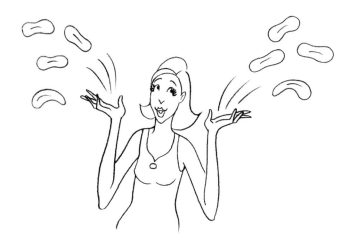

I need to wear a pad

If you wear pads for urinary leakage, make sure they are proper continence pads which are designed to retain urine and prevent odour. If you use your pelvic floor muscles correctly you could soon find that you won't need pads – so keep exercising.

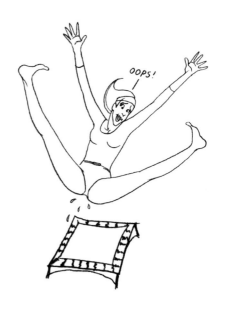

Restrictions for floppy gussets

If your pelvic floor muscles are weak you should avoid high impact sports until you have exercised them properly and they have become stronger. Beware of the downward forces exerted when jogging or bouncing on a trampoline. If your gusset is weak it is asking for trouble. Better to make sure your gusset muscles are fit and strong first.

Restrictions for prolapsed gussets

The front wall or back wall of your vagina may descend and cause you discomfort. This is called a prolapse. Pelvic floor exercises are very helpful for women with mild prolapse. You should definitely avoid heavy lifting. If you feel 'something coming down' and staying down you should visit your GP.

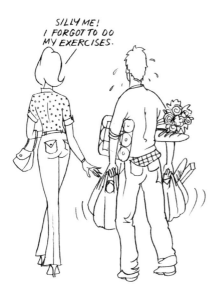

Painful gussets

If you experience discomfort such as stinging or soreness you may have a urinary tract infection and need to visit your GP. If you have pain it may be from pelvic floor muscle spasm. Sometimes the anal sphincter can cramp up and cause very intense pain. Your Specialist Continence Physiotherapist can help you to relax this spasm.

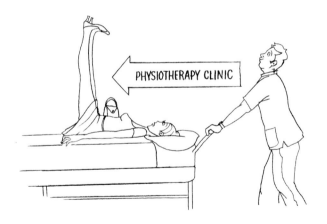

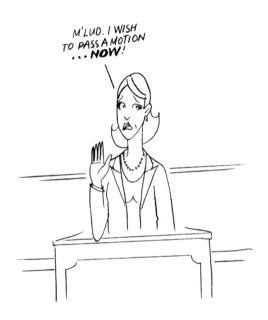

Constipated gussets

Constipation is best avoided. Eat a healthy diet with plenty of fruit and vegetables. Eat breakfast and make time to visit the bathroom before going to work. Never ignore an urge to pass a motion. See your Practice Nurse if you are severely constipated or ask your GP to review any medication you may be taking.

Section 4: Loving your gusset

Washing your gusset

Scented soaps, talcum powder and perfumed sprays are a definite no no when it comes to keeping your gusset clean. They prefer unscented soap and warm, not hot, water. Avoid rubbing the delicate skin, just pat yourself dry and make sure you avoid plastic pants and sheets that cause sweating. If your gusset is itchy you should visit your GP.

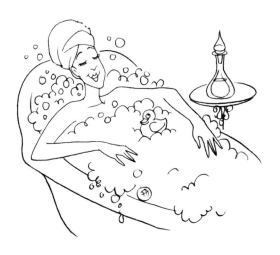

Dress up your gusset

Gussets like to feel special. Treat yourself to some new weekend pants and enjoy that silky feeling. You could even try wearing them in the week. A lot of women feel sexy in G-strings.
Of course you could always go commando. It's a great way of letting your gusset get a little fresh air and it can give your partner a lovely surprise.

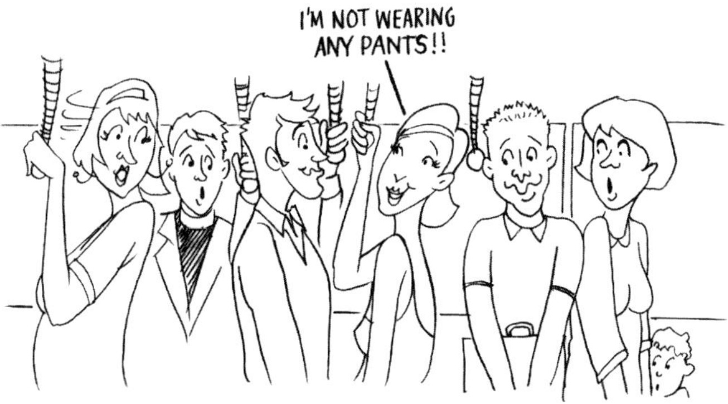
I'M NOT WEARING
ANY PANTS!!

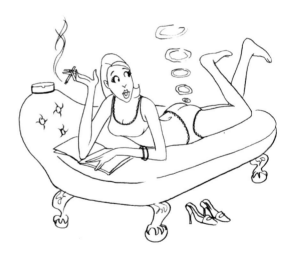

Does smoking affect the health of my gusset?

Yes, smoking causes all the blood vessels in the body to constrict. This can cause your bladder to misbehave. Smoking can cause increased coughing and place extra strain on your gusset. It is an excellent opportunity to start a Smoking Cessation Programme. Your GP will be delighted to give you details.

If I am overweight will my gusset sag more?

Your gusset has to support the weight of your abdominal contents. The more weight you have, the greater the strain on your pelvic floor muscles so it will always help to lose a bit of weight and start doing some pelvic floor exercises.

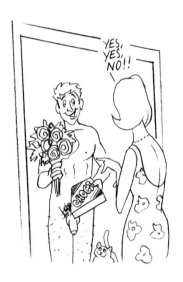

Love your gusset

Every time you tighten your pelvic floor muscles imagine that your gusset is happy and smiling. Imagine that you are the cat who has the cream. Make your gusset smile during sexual activity.

Love your gusset. And your gusset will love you too.

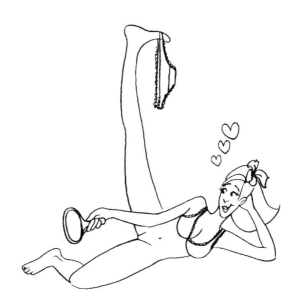

Other books by the same author

All available from www.yourpelvicfloor.co.uk

Clench it or Drench it!
2nd Edition Self-help book for women with urinary leakage
Ed. G Dorey Old Hill Farm, Portmore, Barnstaple, Devon, EX32 0HR, UK
(2006) +44 (0)1271 321 721 £7 + 90p p&p ISBN 0-9545393-1-1

Make it or Fake it!
Self-help book for women with sexual dysfunction
Ed. G Dorey Old Hill Farm, Portmore, Barnstaple, Devon, EX32 0HR, UK
(2003) +44 (0)1271 321 721 £7 + 90p p&p ISBN 0-9545393-0-3

Prevent it!
Guide for men and women with leakage from the back passage
Ed. G Dorey, NEEN Mobilis Healthcare, 100 Shaw Road, Oldham OL1 4AY,
UK (2004) +44 (0)161 925 3180 £7 + 90p p&p ISBN 0-9541445-1-1

Use it or Lose it!
2nd Edition Self-help book for men with urinary leakage and erectile dysfunction
Ed. G Dorey, NEEN Mobilis Healthcare, 100 Shaw Road, Oldham OL1 4AY, UK (2004) +44 (0)161 925 3180 £7 + 90p p&p ISBN 0-9541445-0-3

Living and Loving After Prostate Surgery
Ed. G Dorey Old Hill Farm, Portmore, Barnstaple, Devon, EX32 0HR, UK (2005) +44 (0)1271 321 721 £7 + 90p p&p ISBN 0-9545393-2-X

Stronger and Longer!
Improving erections with pelvic floor exercises
Ed. G Dorey Old Hill Farm, Portmore, Barnstaple, Devon, EX32 0HR, UK (2005) +44 (0)1271 321 721 £7 + 90p p&p ISBN 0-9545393-3-8

Thanks & Links

Expert clinical reviewers:
Kay Crotty MCSP Chartered Physiotherapist
Jennifer Wonnacott MSc BASRT and
UKCP accredited Psychotherapist and
Psychosexual Therapist
Sally Openshaw MSc BASRT accredited
Psychosexual Psychotherapist

Editor: Martin Dorey
www.copymonkey.biz

Design: Tigerplum
www.tigerplum.com

Illustrations by Peter Clover